The Ultimate Renal Diet Cookbook for Seniors

Over 2200 Days of Quick and Delicious

Recipes and a 5-Week Meal Plan for

Optimal Kidney Care

By Unity Demers

Table Of Contents

Chapter 1: Understanding the Renal Diet

The Basics of Kidney Health and Nutrition

Understanding the essentials of kidney health and its interplay with nutrition is akin to exploring a complex dance, where every nutrient and every sip of water plays a part in a finely tuned ballet. These vital organs, often underestimated in their significance, perform a series of crucial functions beyond mere waste filtration. They are the stewards of our body's internal environment, meticulously balancing fluids, electrolytes, and blood pressure. The sustenance we choose has a profound impact on their performance, either supporting their functions or adding to their burden.

Imagine these organs as sophisticated, yet delicate, processing units. Each morsel of food and every drop of liquid we consume passes through their scrutiny. The journey to support their health starts with a conscious choice of foods, focusing not only on their immediate taste or nutritional value but also on their long-term impact on these critical organs.

Proteins, essential for the body's repair and growth, require careful consideration in this context. The type and quantity of protein ingested directly influence their workload. High-protein diets, particularly those rich in animal protein, can exert significant strain on them, especially if their functioning is not optimal. The strategy, therefore, involves balancing quantity with quality – choosing proteins that fulfill bodily needs without overburdening these organs.

Sodium, a common element in our diets, especially prevalent in processed foods, demands cautious management. Its excessive intake can lead to increased blood pressure, challenging their ability to maintain fluid balance. The key is not just reducing the use of table salt but also being vigilant about the hidden sodium in various foods and opting for fresh, minimally processed ingredients.

Phosphorus, though a lesser-discussed mineral, is crucial in this equation. It plays a vital role in bone health, but in the context of reduced functionality, its management becomes essential. Excess phosphorus can have detrimental effects, necessitating a watchful approach to its intake, particularly from certain dairy products, nuts, and processed foods.

Hydration, a fundamental aspect of health, has a unique relationship with these organs. They are responsible for maintaining fluid balance, and thus, understanding individual hydration needs is critical. This involves not only monitoring fluid intake but also being aware of the water content in various foods.

Potassium, vital for several physiological processes, including muscle contractions and nerve function, requires a nuanced approach. Both its excess and deficiency can have serious health implications, underscoring the need for a tailored intake based on individual health and functionality.

Beyond these specific nutrients, the broader dietary pattern plays a significant role. It's about embracing a diet rich in fruits, vegetables, whole grains, and lean proteins, which supports overall health and in turn, aids their functioning. It's also about limiting the intake of certain substances like alcohol and caffeine, which can have adverse effects on blood pressure and hydration levels.

Moreover, the way we approach eating has a substantial impact. Mindful eating – paying attention to what, when, and how much we eat – can go a long way in supporting their health. It's about listening to our body, understanding its cues, and responding with nourishment that is both satisfying and beneficial.

Key Nutrients in the Renal Diet: What to Watch

Navigating the landscape of a renal diet involves a keen understanding of various nutrients and their roles in supporting the body's filtration system. This diet is more than just a list of do's and don'ts; it's a nuanced approach to nutrition that respects and aids the body's natural balancing act.

Proteins, vital for bodily repairs and functions, require thoughtful consideration in this context. The quantity and quality of protein consumed directly impact the workload of the body's filters. Animal proteins, high in phosphorus and potentially burdensome, call for moderation. Plant-based proteins emerge as a kidney-gentler alternative, offering essential amino acids without excessive strain.

Sodium, a ubiquitous dietary component, demands special attention. Excessive intake can lead to fluid retention and elevated blood pressure, posing a challenge to the body's delicate balance. The art of sodium management extends beyond mere salt reduction; it involves a comprehensive understanding of its presence in foods and a shift towards fresh, minimally processed ingredients.

Phosphorus, crucial for bone health and energy, needs careful monitoring, especially when the body's filtering efficiency is compromised. Phosphorus, often lurking unnoticed in processed foods, can accumulate and lead to health complications. The approach here is not to eliminate phosphorus but to be aware of its sources and maintain a balanced intake.

Potassium, essential for various physiological functions, requires a balanced approach. The body's ability to regulate potassium levels can be affected in cases of reduced renal efficiency, making individualized intake recommendations crucial. Both its excess and deficiency can pose health risks, underscoring the need for tailored dietary adjustments.

Calcium's interplay with phosphorus and its role in bone health make it a nutrient of interest. Ensuring adequate calcium intake, without going overboard, is essential in managing the phosphorus-calcium balance, especially when phosphorus intake needs to be controlled.

Fluids play a critical role in kidney health. The right balance of fluid intake is essential, as these organs regulate the body's fluid levels. This balance, however, is not uniform for everyone. It varies based on individual health, lifestyle, and specific renal function.

Iron is vital, particularly as anemia is a common concern in renal health. The diet needs to ensure adequate iron intake to prevent anemia, yet the absorption and utilization of iron can be complex in renal conditions, necessitating a nuanced approach to its inclusion in the diet.

Vitamins, specifically water-soluble ones like vitamin C, and fat-soluble ones like vitamins D and A, are important in a renal diet. The body's ability to process and utilize these vitamins can be affected by renal health, making it important to tailor their intake accordingly.

Adapting Your Lifestyle for Kidney Health

Adopting a lifestyle that supports renal health is a multifaceted endeavor, transcending beyond mere dietary adjustments. It encompasses a holistic approach, where every aspect of daily living is aligned to nurture and protect these vital organs.

The cornerstone of this adapted lifestyle is mindful nutrition. Embracing a renal-friendly diet is about making informed choices in what to eat and drink. This involves not just selecting the right foods but also understanding portion sizes and the nutritional content of meals. Planning meals thoughtfully ensures that the diet remains rich in essential nutrients while being gentle on these organs.

Physical activity, a key player in overall well-being, plays a significant role in supporting renal health. Regular, moderate exercise aids in controlling blood pressure, maintaining a healthy weight, and enhancing cardiovascular health, all of which are beneficial for these organs. The choice of activity should resonate with personal preferences, ensuring sustainability and enjoyment, be it walking, swimming, cycling, or yoga.

Hydration is a delicate balance in a renal-conscious lifestyle. These organs play a crucial role in managing the body's fluid levels, so understanding individual hydration needs is essential. The right amount of fluid intake supports their function without overburdening them. This involves not just monitoring water intake but also being cognizant of the fluid content in various foods.

Managing stress is another vital component. Chronic stress can adversely affect overall health, including renal well-being. Incorporating stress-reduction techniques like meditation, deep breathing exercises, or engaging in relaxing hobbies helps in mitigating its negative impact.

Sleep quality has a direct correlation with renal health. Adequate, restful sleep is vital for the body's healing and regeneration processes. Maintaining a consistent sleep schedule and ensuring a comfortable, restful sleeping environment are key to fostering good sleep hygiene.

Medication management is particularly crucial for those with existing renal concerns. Certain medications can have implications on these organs, so regular consultations with healthcare providers for medication reviews are imperative. This ensures that any medication regimen is aligned with individual health needs and doesn't inadvertently compromise renal function.

Regular health screenings play a critical role in a renal-conscious lifestyle. Monitoring renal function and overall health through periodic check-ups aids in early detection and management of potential issues. Being proactive about health checks underscores a commitment to maintaining renal well-being.

Emotional well-being is integral to this lifestyle adaptation. Building and nurturing a support system provides emotional resilience. Sharing experiences and challenges with others who understand the journey can be immensely comforting and empowering.

Chapter 2: Breakfasts to Start Your Day

Quick and Nutritious Smoothies

Berry Almond Bliss

- **P.T.:** 10 mins
- **Ingr.:** 1 cup mixed berries (blueberries, strawberries, raspberries), 1/2 banana, 2 tbsp almond butter, 1 cup almond milk, 1 tsp chia seeds, 1 tsp honey (optional).
- **Procedure:** Blend all ingredients until smooth. Adjust consistency with additional almond milk if needed.
- **Tips:** Use frozen berries for a thicker smoothie. Add a scoop of whey protein for an extra protein boost.
- **N.I.:** Rich in antioxidants, low in phosphorus and potassium, with a good balance of protein and healthy fats.

Green Detoxifier

- **P.T.:** 8 mins
- **Ingr.:** 1 cup spinach, 1/2 green apple, 1/2 cucumber, 1 tbsp flaxseed, 1 cup coconut water, juice of 1/2 lemon.
- **Procedure:** Combine all ingredients in a blender and puree until smooth.
- **Tips:** Add a few mint leaves for added freshness. Ideal for a morning detox.
- **N.I.:** Low in sodium and potassium, high in fiber and vitamins A and C.

Tropical Turmeric Tango

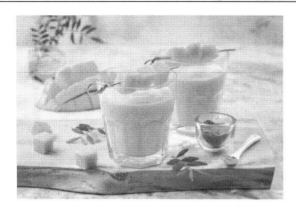

- **P.T.:** 10 mins
- **Ingr.:** 1/2 cup pineapple chunks, 1/2 mango, 1/2 tsp turmeric powder, 1 cup rice milk, 1 tsp grated ginger, 1 tbsp honey.

- **Procedure:** Blend all ingredients until smooth, ensuring the turmeric is well incorporated.
- **Tips:** Use ripe mango for natural sweetness.
  Great anti-inflammatory properties.
- **N.I.:** Good source of vitamin C, low in phosphorus, with anti-inflammatory benefits.

Protein Power Punch

- **P.T.:** 10 mins
- **Ingr.:** 1/2 cup cottage cheese (low sodium), 1/4 cup rolled oats, 1/2 banana, 1 tbsp almond butter, 1 cup oat milk, a dash of cinnamon.

- **Procedure:** Blend until smooth. Add water to adjust consistency.
- **Tips:** Ideal post-workout smoothie. Can add a scoop of protein powder for extra protein.
- **N.I.:** High in protein, moderate in potassium, low in sodium.

Avocado Zen Blend

- **P.T.:** 10 mins
- **Ingr.:** 1/2 ripe avocado, 1 cup spinach, 1/2 pear, 1 tbsp chia seeds, 1 cup hemp milk, a dash of vanilla extract.
- **Procedure:** Puree all ingredients until creamy and smooth.
- **Tips:** Add a few drops of stevia for a sweeter taste. Perfect for a filling breakfast.
- **N.I.:** High in healthy fats, fiber, low in sodium and potassium.

Low-Phosphorus Pancakes and Waffles

Oat and Almond Flour Pancakes

- **P.T.:** 15 mins
- **Ingr.:** 1 cup oat flour, 1/2 cup almond flour, 1 tsp baking powder (aluminum-free), 1 egg, 1 cup almond milk, 1 tbsp honey, a pinch of salt.
- **Procedure:** Mix dry ingredients. Whisk in egg, almond milk, and honey. Cook on a non-stick skillet until golden.
- **Tips:** Serve with fresh berries or a light drizzle of maple syrup.
- **N.I.:** Low in phosphorus and sodium, high in fiber.

Banana Chia Waffles

- **P.T.:** 20 mins
- **Ingr.:** 1 mashed banana, 2 tbsp chia seeds, 1 cup whole wheat flour, 1/2 tsp baking powder, 1 cup rice milk, 1 tsp vanilla extract.
- **Procedure:** Combine ingredients to form a batter. Cook in a preheated waffle iron until crispy.
- **Tips:** Chia seeds add a nice crunch and are a great source of omega-3s.
- **N.I.:** Rich in omega-3 fatty acids, low in phosphorus.

Buckwheat and Blueberry Pancakes

- **P.T.:** 18 mins
- **Ingr.:** 1 cup buckwheat flour, 1 cup almond milk, 1/2 cup blueberries, 1 egg, 1 tbsp maple syrup, 1/2 tsp baking soda.
- **Procedure:** Mix ingredients to create batter. Pour scoops onto a hot griddle, flipping once bubbles form.
- **Tips:** Buckwheat flour gives a robust flavor and pairs well with blueberries.
- **N.I.:** High in antioxidants, low in sodium and phosphorus.

Quinoa Flour Waffles

- **P.T.:** 25 mins
- **Ingr.:** 1 cup quinoa flour, 1 tsp baking powder, 1 cup oat milk, 2 eggs, 1 tbsp melted coconut oil, 1 tsp cinnamon.
- **Procedure:** Mix wet and dry ingredients separately, then combine. Cook in a waffle iron until golden.
- **Tips:** Quinoa flour adds a unique, nutty flavor to the waffles.
- **N.I.:** Good source of protein, low in phosphorus.

Sweet Potato and Flaxseed Pancakes

- **P.T.:** 20 mins
- **Ingr.:** 1 cup mashed sweet potato, 2 tbsp ground flaxseed, 1 cup rice flour, 1/2 tsp baking powder, 1 cup hemp milk, 1 tsp nutmeg.
- **Procedure:** Combine all ingredients. Pour batter onto a heated skillet and cook until fluffy.
- **Tips:** Sweet potato adds natural sweetness and moistness to the pancakes.
- **N.I.:** High in fiber, low in sodium, and rich in beta-carotene.

Kidney-Friendly Egg Dishes

Herbed Veggie Scramble

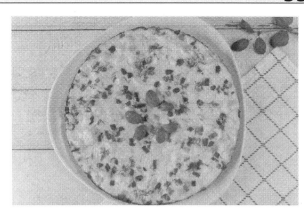

- **P.T.:** 12 mins

- **Ingr.:** 2 eggs, 1/4 cup diced bell peppers, 1/4 cup chopped spinach, 1 tbsp chopped chives, 1 tbsp olive oil, salt and pepper to taste.
- **Procedure:** Sauté veggies in olive oil. Add beaten eggs and cook until set. Garnish with chives.
- **Tips:** Use a variety of colorful veggies for an appealing dish.
- **N.I.:** High in protein, low in potassium and phosphorus.

Mediterranean Frittata

- **P.T.:** 20 mins
- **Ingr.:** 4 eggs, 1/2 cup diced tomatoes, 1/4 cup sliced olives, 1/4 cup feta cheese, 1 tbsp parsley, 1 tsp olive oil.

- **Procedure:** Sauté tomatoes and olives in oil. Pour beaten eggs over. Sprinkle with feta and bake until set.
- **Tips:** Serve with a side of mixed greens.
- **N.I.:** Moderate in phosphorus, low in sodium, rich in healthy fats.

Avocado Egg Cups

- **P.T.:** 30 mins
- **Ingr.:** 2 avocados, halved and pitted, 4 eggs, salt, pepper, and paprika to taste.
- **Procedure:** Place avocado halves in a baking dish. Crack an egg into each. Bake until eggs are set.
- **Tips:** Perfect for a high-energy breakfast. Garnish with paprika for extra flavor.
- **N.I.:** High in healthy fats, low in sodium.

Spinach and Mushroom Omelette

- **P.T.:** 15 mins
- **Ingr.:** 3 eggs, 1/2 cup sliced mushrooms, 1/2 cup spinach, 1 tbsp grated Parmesan, 1 tsp olive oil.
- **Procedure:** Sauté mushrooms and spinach. Pour beaten eggs over veggies, cook until set, fold, and top with Parmesan.
- **Tips:** Add fresh herbs for more flavor.
- **N.I.:** High in protein and iron, low in phosphorus.

Egg and Quinoa Breakfast Bowl

- **P.T.:** 25 mins
- **Ingr.:** 1/2 cup cooked quinoa, 2 poached eggs, 1/4 cup diced avocado, 1 tbsp pumpkin seeds, salt, and pepper to taste.
- **Procedure:** Place quinoa in a bowl, top with poached eggs, avocado, and pumpkin seeds.
- **Tips:** Season with herbs for added flavor. Ideal for a post-workout meal.
- **N.I.:** Balanced in protein and carbs, low in sodium, rich in healthy fats.

Chapter 3: Light and Refreshing Salads

Greens and Kidney Health: Choosing the Best

Crisp Arugula and Apple Salad

- **P.T.:** 10 mins
- **Ingr.:** 2 cups arugula, 1 sliced green apple, 1/4 cup walnut halves, 2 tbsp crumbled goat cheese, dressing (olive oil, lemon juice, Dijon mustard).

- **Procedure:** Toss arugula, apple, and walnuts with dressing. Top with goat cheese.
- **Tips:** Dress the salad right before serving to keep the arugula crisp.
- **N.I.:** Low in potassium, high in vitamin K and fiber.

Refreshing Cucumber and Dill Salad

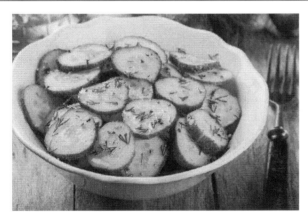

- **P.T.:** 15 mins
- **Ingr.:** 2 medium cucumbers (thinly sliced), 2 tbsp chopped dill, 1/4 red onion (thinly sliced), dressing (white wine vinegar, a touch of honey, olive oil).

- **Procedure:** Combine cucumbers, dill, and onion. Drizzle with dressing and toss gently.
- **Tips:** Let it chill for an hour before serving for enhanced flavors.
- **N.I.:** Low in sodium and phosphorus, refreshing and hydrating.

Spinach and Strawberry Sensation

- **P.T.:** 10 mins
- **Ingr.:** 2 cups baby spinach, 1 cup sliced strawberries, 1/4 cup sliced almonds, dressing (balsamic vinegar, olive oil, black pepper).
- **Procedure:** Toss spinach with strawberries and almonds. Add dressing and mix.
- **Tips:** Use fresh, ripe strawberries for natural sweetness.
- **N.I.:** Rich in antioxidants, low in potassium.

Mixed Greens with Roasted Beetroot

- **P.T.:** 45 mins (includes roasting)
- **Ingr.:** 2 cups mixed greens (lettuce, arugula), 2 roasted beetroots (cubed), 2 tbsp pumpkin seeds, dressing (apple cider vinegar, olive oil, mustard).
- **Procedure:** Toss greens with beetroot and pumpkin seeds. Drizzle dressing over salad.
- **Tips:** Roast extra beetroot for future use; it keeps well in the fridge.
- **N.I.:** High in fiber, low in sodium, good for blood pressure management.

Kale and Avocado Delight

- **P.T.:** 12 mins
- **Ingr.:** 2 cups chopped kale, 1 ripe avocado (cubed), 1/4 cup sunflower seeds, dressing (lemon juice, olive oil, minced garlic).
- **Procedure:** Massage kale with dressing, then mix in avocado and sunflower seeds.
- **Tips:** Massaging kale softens its texture and enhances taste.
- **N.I.:** Rich in healthy fats, low in phosphorus, nutrient-dense.

Protein-Packed Salads for Energy

Tofu and Edamame Salad Bowl

- **P.T.:** 20 mins
- **Ingr.:** 1 cup diced firm tofu, 1/2 cup edamame, 2 cups mixed greens, 1/4 cup shredded carrots, dressing (low-sodium soy sauce, sesame oil, rice vinegar).
- **Procedure:** Toss tofu and edamame with greens and carrots. Drizzle with dressing.
- **Tips:** Marinate tofu in soy sauce mixture for extra flavor.
- **N.I.:** High in plant protein, low in phosphorus and sodium.

Chickpea and Avocado Medley

- **P.T.:** 15 mins
- **Ingr.:** 1 cup cooked chickpeas, 1 ripe avocado (cubed), 2 cups arugula, 1/4 cup diced red onion, dressing (lemon juice, olive oil, minced garlic).
- **Procedure:** Combine all ingredients and toss gently with dressing.
- **Tips:** Chill for 30 minutes before serving for enhanced flavors.
- **N.I.:** Rich in fiber and healthy fats, low in potassium.

Grilled Chicken and Quinoa Salad

- **P.T.:** 30 mins
- **Ingr.:** 1/2 cup cooked quinoa, 1 grilled chicken breast (sliced), 2 cups baby spinach, 1/4 cup cherry tomatoes (halved), dressing (balsamic vinegar, Dijon mustard, olive oil).
- **Procedure:** Mix quinoa, chicken, spinach, and tomatoes. Top with dressing.
- **Tips:** Grill extra chicken for a quick protein addition to any meal.
- **N.I.:** Balanced in protein and carbs, low in sodium.

Salmon and Kale Caesar

- **P.T.:** 25 mins
- **Ingr.:** 1 grilled salmon fillet, 2 cups chopped kale, 2 tbsp grated Parmesan cheese, dressing (low-fat Greek yogurt, lemon juice, Worcestershire sauce).
- **Procedure:** Toss kale in dressing, top with salmon and Parmesan.
- **Tips:** Massage kale with dressing to soften leaves.
- **N.I.:** High in omega-3 fatty acids, low in phosphorus.

Lentil and Roasted Veggie Toss

- **P.T.:** 40 mins
- **Ingr.:** 1 cup cooked lentils, 1 cup roasted vegetables (zucchini, bell pepper), 2 cups mixed greens, dressing (red wine vinegar, olive oil, minced mint).
- **Procedure:** Combine lentils, roasted veggies, and greens. Add dressing.
- **Tips:** Roast extra veggies for an easy meal addition.
- **N.I.:** High in plant-based protein, rich in vitamins and minerals, low in sodium.

Dressings and Toppings: Flavor without Harm

Lemon Herb Vinaigrette

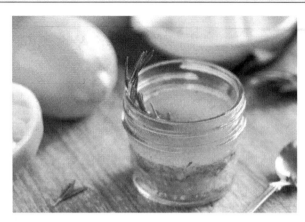

- **P.T.:** 5 mins

- **Ingr.:** 1/4 cup olive oil, 2 tbsp fresh lemon juice, 1 tsp Dijon mustard, 1 tbsp chopped fresh herbs (parsley, basil), black pepper to taste.
- **Procedure:** Whisk all ingredients until emulsified.
- **Tips:** Store in a jar and shake well before each use.
- **N.I.:** Low in sodium, rich in antioxidants.

Creamy Avocado Dressing

- **P.T.:** 10 mins
- **Ingr.:** 1 ripe avocado, 1/4 cup Greek yogurt, 1 tbsp lime juice, 1 clove garlic (minced), water to thin.
- **Procedure:** Blend all ingredients until smooth, adding water as needed for consistency.
- **Tips:** Perfect for drizzling over hearty salads or as a dip.
- **N.I.:** High in healthy fats, low in potassium.

Raspberry Walnut Vinaigrette

- **P.T.:** 10 mins
- **Ingr.:** 1/4 cup raspberry puree, 2 tbsp walnut oil, 1 tbsp white wine vinegar, 1 tsp honey, salt and pepper to taste.
- **Procedure:** Blend all ingredients until smooth.
- **Tips:** Use fresh raspberries for the puree for extra freshness.
- **N.I.:** Low in phosphorus, rich in omega-3 fatty acids.

Cilantro Lime Dressing

- **P.T.:** 7 mins
- **Ingr.:** 1/4 cup chopped cilantro, 1/4 cup olive oil, juice of 2 limes, 1 tsp honey, 1 small jalapeño (seeded, optional).
- **Procedure:** Puree all ingredients in a blender.
- **Tips:** Adjust the amount of jalapeño for desired heat.
- **N.I.:** Low in sodium, adds a zesty flavor to salads.

Toasted Sesame Ginger Dressing

- **P.T.:** 10 mins
- **Ingr.:** 2 tbsp toasted sesame oil, 1 tbsp grated ginger, 2 tbsp low-sodium soy sauce, 1 tbsp rice vinegar, 1 tsp honey.
- **Procedure:** Whisk together all ingredients until well combined.
- **Tips:** Great for Asian-inspired salads or as a marinade.
- **N.I.:** Low in potassium, high in flavor.

Chapter 4: Soups and Stews

Comforting Broths and Soups

Carrot and Ginger Puree Soup

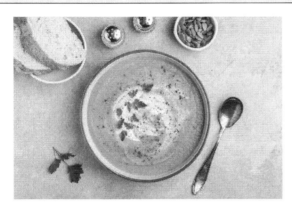

- **P.T.:** 30 mins
- **Ingr.:** 4 large carrots (peeled and chopped), 1 tbsp grated ginger, 1 onion (chopped), 4 cups vegetable broth (low sodium), 1 tbsp olive oil, salt and pepper to taste.

- **Procedure:** Sauté onion and ginger in olive oil, add carrots, pour in broth. Simmer until carrots are tender. Puree until smooth.
- **Tips:** Garnish with a dollop of Greek yogurt for creaminess.
- **N.I.:** Low in sodium, high in vitamin A and antioxidants.

Lentil and Spinach Broth

- **P.T.:** 45 mins
- **Ingr.:** 1 cup red lentils, 2 cups spinach, 1 diced carrot, 1 diced celery stalk, 5 cups vegetable broth (low sodium), 1 tsp cumin, 1 tbsp olive oil.

- **Procedure:** Cook lentils, carrot, and celery in broth. Add spinach and cumin in the last 5 minutes.
- **Tips:** Serve with a slice of whole-grain bread for a hearty meal.
- **N.I.:** Rich in plant-based protein, low in potassium.

Tomato Basil Soup

- **P.T.:** 25 mins
- **Ingr.:** 4 cups chopped tomatoes, 2 tbsp fresh basil (chopped), 1 onion (chopped), 3 cups vegetable broth (low sodium), 1 tbsp olive oil, garlic powder to taste.
- **Procedure:** Sauté onion, add tomatoes and broth. Simmer and add basil. Blend until smooth.
- **Tips:** Add a touch of cream for richness, if desired.
- **N.I.:** Low in phosphorus, high in lycopene.

Mushroom and Barley Soup

- **P.T.:** 50 mins
- **Ingr.:** 1 cup sliced mushrooms, 1/2 cup barley, 1 diced onion, 4 cups vegetable broth (low sodium), 1 tsp thyme, 1 tbsp olive oil.
- **Procedure:** Sauté mushrooms and onion, add barley and broth. Cook until barley is tender.
- **Tips:** Perfect for a cozy evening meal.
- **N.I.:** High in fiber, low in sodium.

Butternut Squash and Apple Soup

- **P.T.:** 40 mins
- **Ingr.:** 2 cups butternut squash (cubed), 1 apple (peeled and chopped), 1 onion (chopped), 4 cups vegetable broth (low sodium), 1 tsp cinnamon, 1 tbsp olive oil.
- **Procedure:** Sauté onion, add squash and apple, pour in broth. Cook until soft. Blend until smooth.
- **Tips:** Garnish with a sprinkle of cinnamon.
- **N.I.:** Low in potassium, rich in vitamins.

Hearty Stews for All Seasons

Winter Vegetable and Bean Stew

- **P.T.:** 1 hour
- **Ingr.:** 2 cups low-sodium vegetable broth, 1 cup chopped carrots, 1 cup chopped parsnips, 1 cup white beans (soaked and drained), 1 onion (diced), 2 cloves garlic (minced), 1 tsp thyme, 1 tbsp olive oil.
- **Procedure:** Sauté onion and garlic in olive oil. Add vegetables, beans, thyme, and broth. Simmer until vegetables are tender.
- **Tips:** Serve with a sprinkle of fresh parsley for added flavor.
- **N.I.:** High in fiber, low in sodium, rich in plant-based protein.

Hearty Chicken and Barley Stew

- **P.T.:** 50 mins
- **Ingr.:** 1 lb chicken breast (cubed), 1/2 cup barley, 4 cups low-sodium chicken broth, 1 cup diced carrots, 1 cup diced celery, 1 tsp rosemary, 1 tbsp olive oil.
- **Procedure:** Brown chicken in olive oil. Add vegetables, barley, rosemary, and broth. Simmer until barley is tender.
- **Tips:** Shred the chicken for a different texture.
- **N.I.:** Low in potassium, high in protein.

Moroccan Lentil and Vegetable Stew

- **P.T.:** 1 hour
- **Ingr.:** 1 cup green lentils, 1 can diced tomatoes, 1 cup chopped zucchini, 1 cup diced butternut squash, 4 cups low-sodium vegetable broth, 1 tsp cumin, 1 tsp paprika, 1 tbsp olive oil.
- **Procedure:** Sauté spices in oil, add vegetables, lentils, tomatoes, and broth. Simmer until lentils are cooked.
- **Tips:** Garnish with lemon zest for a fresh taste.
- **N.I.:** High in fiber, low in sodium, rich in nutrients.

Beef and Mushroom Stew

- **P.T.:** 1 hour 30 mins
- **Ingr.:** 1 lb lean beef (cubed), 2 cups sliced mushrooms, 4 cups low-sodium beef broth, 1 cup diced potatoes, 1 onion (chopped), 1 tsp thyme, 1 tbsp olive oil.
- **Procedure:** Brown beef in olive oil, add onions, mushrooms, potatoes, thyme, and broth. Simmer until beef is tender.
- **Tips:** Thickening the stew with a bit of cornstarch can give it a heartier texture.
- **N.I.:** Rich in protein, low in phosphorus.

Spicy Tomato and Chickpea Stew

- **P.T.:** 40 mins
- **Ingr.:** 1 can chickpeas (drained and rinsed), 1 can diced tomatoes, 1 diced bell pepper, 1 diced onion, 4 cups low-sodium vegetable broth, 1 tsp cayenne pepper, 1 tsp cumin, 1 tbsp olive oil.
- **Procedure:** Sauté onion and bell pepper in olive oil, add spices, chickpeas, tomatoes, and broth. Simmer for 30 minutes.
- **Tips:** Adjust the amount of cayenne to control the heat.
- **N.I.:** High in plant-based protein, low in sodium, rich in flavor.

Managing Sodium in Homemade Soups

Garden Fresh Vegetable Soup

- **P.T.:** 35 mins
- **Ingr.:** 2 cups chopped mixed vegetables (carrots, zucchini, bell peppers), 1 onion (diced), 3 cups low-sodium vegetable broth, 1 tsp dried basil, 1 tbsp olive oil.
- **Procedure:** Sauté onion in olive oil, add vegetables, basil, and broth. Simmer until vegetables are tender.
- **Tips:** Add a squeeze of fresh lemon juice before serving for a zesty twist.
- **N.I.:** Low in sodium, high in vitamins and minerals.

Creamy Cauliflower and Garlic Soup

- **P.T.:** 40 mins
- **Ingr.:** 1 head cauliflower (chopped), 4 cloves garlic (minced), 4 cups low-sodium vegetable broth, 1/2 cup almond milk, 1 tsp thyme, 1 tbsp olive oil.
- **Procedure:** Roast cauliflower and garlic. Blend with broth, almond milk, and thyme until smooth.
- **Tips:** Garnish with roasted pumpkin seeds for a crunchy texture.
- **N.I.:** Low in phosphorus and sodium, rich in antioxidants.

Butternut Squash and Lentil Soup

- **P.T.:** 50 mins
- **Ingr.:** 2 cups butternut squash (cubed), 1 cup red lentils, 1 onion (chopped), 4 cups low-sodium vegetable broth, 1 tsp cumin, 1 tbsp olive oil.
- **Procedure:** Sauté onion, add squash, lentils, cumin, and broth. Cook until lentils are soft.
- **Tips:** Blend for a smoother texture, if preferred.
- **N.I.:** High in fiber, low in sodium, good source of plant protein.

Spicy Tomato and Chickpea Soup

- **P.T.:** 30 mins
- **Ingr.:** 1 can chickpeas (drained and rinsed), 1 can no-salt-added diced tomatoes, 1 onion (chopped), 1 red bell pepper (chopped), 4 cups low-sodium vegetable broth, 1 tsp smoked paprika, 1 tbsp olive oil.
- **Procedure:** Sauté onion and bell pepper, add tomatoes, chickpeas, paprika, and broth. Simmer for 20 mins.
- **Tips:** Add fresh cilantro for a burst of flavor.
- **N.I.:** Low in sodium, high in protein and fiber.

Chapter 5: Main Course: Vegetarian Delights

Plant-Based Proteins: A Kidney-Friendly Guide

Quinoa and Black Bean Bowl

- **P.T.:** 25 mins
- **Ingr.:** 1 cup cooked quinoa, 1/2 cup black beans (low sodium, drained), 1/2 cup corn, 1 diced bell pepper, dressing (lime juice, olive oil, cumin).
- **Procedure:** Combine quinoa, beans, corn, and pepper. Drizzle with dressing.
- **Tips:** Top with avocado slices for extra creaminess.
- **N.I.:** High in plant protein, low in sodium and potassium.

Tofu and Broccoli Stir-Fry

- **P.T.:** 20 mins
- **Ingr.:** 1 block firm tofu (cubed), 2 cups broccoli florets, 1 onion (sliced), 2 cloves garlic (minced), sauce (low-sodium soy sauce, ginger, sesame oil).
- **Procedure:** Sauté tofu until golden, add vegetables and sauce. Cook until broccoli is tender.
- **Tips:** Serve over brown rice or whole grain noodles.
- **N.I.:** Rich in protein, low in phosphorus.

Lentil Stuffed Bell Peppers

- **P.T.:** 45 mins
- **Ingr.:** 4 bell peppers (halved), 1 cup cooked lentils, 1 diced tomato, 1 diced onion, 1 tsp smoked paprika, 1 tbsp olive oil.
- **Procedure:** Sauté onion, mix in lentils, tomato, paprika. Stuff peppers, bake until tender.
- **Tips:** Sprinkle with nutritional yeast for a cheesy flavor.
- **N.I.:** High in fiber, low in sodium, kidney-friendly.

Chickpea and Spinach Curry

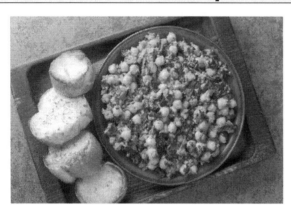

- **P.T.:** 30 mins
- **Ingr.:** 1 can chickpeas (drained, rinsed), 2 cups spinach, 1 can diced tomatoes, 1 onion (chopped), 1 tbsp curry powder, 1 tbsp olive oil.
- **Procedure:** Sauté onion, add chickpeas, tomatoes, spinach, and curry. Simmer until thickened.
- **Tips:** Serve with a side of basmati rice.
- **N.I.:** Low in potassium, high in plant-based protein.

Eggplant and Mushroom Ragout

- **P.T.:** 40 mins
- **Ingr.:** 1 large eggplant (cubed), 2 cups mushrooms (sliced), 1 can no-salt-added diced tomatoes, 1 onion (chopped), 1 clove garlic (minced), 1 tsp oregano, 1 tbsp olive oil.
- **Procedure:** Sauté onion, garlic, add eggplant, mushrooms, tomatoes, oregano. Simmer until eggplant is tender.
- **Tips:** Excellent when topped with fresh basil.
- **N.I.:** Low in sodium and phosphorus, rich in antioxidants.

Flavorful Vegetable Stir-Fries and Curries

Coconut Veggie Stir-Fry

- **P.T.:** 20 mins
- **Ingr.:** 2 cups mixed vegetables (broccoli, bell pepper, carrot), 1 can coconut milk, 1 tbsp coconut oil, 1 tsp turmeric, 1 tbsp low-sodium soy sauce, 1 tsp grated ginger.
- **Procedure:** Sauté vegetables in coconut oil, add turmeric and ginger. Stir in coconut milk and soy sauce. Cook until veggies are tender.
- **Tips:** Serve over jasmine rice for a complete meal.
- **N.I.:** Low in sodium, rich in antioxidants.

Spiced Chickpea Curry

- **P.T.:** 30 mins
- **Ingr.:** 1 can chickpeas (drained, rinsed), 2 cups spinach, 1 diced tomato, 1 onion (chopped), 1 tsp garam masala, 1 tbsp olive oil, 1 cup low-sodium vegetable broth.
- **Procedure:** Sauté onion, add garam masala, tomato, chickpeas, broth. Simmer, then add spinach.
- **Tips:** Garnish with cilantro for a fresh flavor.
- **N.I.:** High in fiber, low in potassium.

Tofu and Green Bean Stir-Fry

- **P.T.:** 25 mins
- **Ingr.:** 1 block firm tofu (cubed), 2 cups green beans, 1 bell pepper (sliced), 1 tbsp sesame oil, sauce (2 tbsp low-sodium soy sauce, 1 tsp honey, 1 tsp garlic powder).
- **Procedure:** Sauté tofu in sesame oil until golden. Add vegetables and sauce. Cook until beans are tender.
- **Tips:** Add a sprinkle of sesame seeds before serving.
- **N.I.:** Rich in plant protein, low in phosphorus.

Eggplant and Lentil Curry

- **P.T.:** 40 mins
- **Ingr.:** 1 large eggplant (cubed), 1 cup red lentils, 1 can diced tomatoes, 1 onion (chopped), 1 tsp cumin, 1 tbsp coconut oil, 1 cup low-sodium vegetable broth.
- **Procedure:** Sauté onion and cumin in oil. Add eggplant, lentils, tomatoes, and broth. Simmer until lentils are cooked.
- **Tips:** Serve with a dollop of yogurt for creaminess.
- **N.I.:** High in fiber, low in sodium.

Cauliflower and Pea Stir-Fry

- **P.T.:** 20 mins
- **Ingr.:** 2 cups cauliflower florets, 1 cup frozen peas, 1 red bell pepper (sliced), 1 tbsp olive oil, sauce (1 tsp curry powder, 2 tbsp low-sodium soy sauce, 1 tsp ginger paste).
- **Procedure:** Sauté cauliflower and bell pepper in oil. Add peas, curry powder, soy sauce, and ginger. Cook until veggies are tender.
- **Tips:** Garnish with fresh coriander leaves.
- **N.I.:** Low in potassium, high in vitamin C.

Hearty Vegetarian Casseroles

Quinoa and Vegetable Bake

- **P.T.:** 50 mins
- **Ingr.:** 1 cup quinoa, 2 cups mixed vegetables (zucchini, bell peppers, carrots), 1 can diced tomatoes, 1 tsp Italian herbs, 1/2 cup low-fat cheese, 1 tbsp olive oil.
- **Procedure:** Cook quinoa as directed. Sauté vegetables, mix with quinoa, tomatoes, and herbs. Bake topped with cheese until golden.
- **Tips:** Add a sprinkle of nutritional yeast for extra flavor.
- **N.I.:** Rich in protein, low in sodium and phosphorus.

Broccoli and Cauliflower Gratin

- **P.T.:** 35 mins
- **Ingr.:** 2 cups broccoli florets, 2 cups cauliflower florets, 1/4 cup whole wheat breadcrumbs, 1/2 cup low-fat cheese, sauce (1 cup low-fat milk, 2 tbsp flour, 1 tbsp butter).
- **Procedure:** Steam broccoli and cauliflower. Make a roux with butter and flour, add milk to form a sauce. Combine with vegetables, top with breadcrumbs and cheese, bake until bubbly.
- **Tips:** Broil for the last few minutes for a crispy top.
- **N.I.:** High in calcium, low in potassium.

Sweet Potato and Black Bean Casserole

- **P.T.:** 1 hour
- **Ingr.:** 2 medium sweet potatoes (sliced), 1 cup black beans (low sodium, drained), 1 diced onion, 1 tsp cumin, 1/2 cup low-fat cheese, 1 tbsp olive oil.
- **Procedure:** Layer sweet potatoes, onions, and beans in a dish. Sprinkle cumin, top with cheese. Bake until potatoes are tender.
- **Tips:** Serve with a side of green salad for a complete meal.
- **N.I.:** High in fiber, low in sodium.

Mushroom and Pea Risotto Bake

- **P.T.:** 1 hour
- **Ingr.:** 1 cup Arborio rice, 2 cups sliced mushrooms, 1 cup frozen peas, 1 onion (chopped), 4 cups low-sodium vegetable broth, 1/2 cup grated Parmesan cheese, 1 tbsp olive oil.
- **Procedure:** Sauté onion, add rice and mushrooms, gradually add broth, stirring until absorbed. Add peas, bake with cheese until creamy.
- **Tips:** Garnish with fresh parsley.
- **N.I.:** Low in phosphorus, high in umami flavor.

Zucchini and Tomato Lasagna

- **P.T.:** 1 hour 15 mins
- **Ingr.:** 3 large zucchinis (sliced lengthwise), 2 cups crushed tomatoes, 1 cup ricotta cheese, 1 egg, 1 tsp garlic powder, 1 tbsp olive oil, 1/2 cup low-fat mozzarella.
- **Procedure:** Grill zucchini slices. Mix ricotta with egg and garlic. Layer zucchini, ricotta, tomatoes, and repeat. Top with mozzarella, bake until bubbly.
- **Tips:** Let it sit for 10 minutes before serving to set.
- **N.I.:** High in protein, low in carbohydrates.

Chapter 6: Main Course: Poultry and Meat

Safe Meat Choices for Kidney Health

Grilled Lemon-Herb Chicken

- **P.T.:** 30 mins
- **Ingr.:** 2 chicken breasts, 1 tbsp olive oil, juice of 1 lemon, 1 tsp dried herbs (thyme, oregano), black pepper to taste.
- **Procedure:** Marinate chicken in olive oil, lemon juice, herbs, and pepper. Grill until cooked through.
- **Tips:** Serve with a side of roasted vegetables.
- **N.I.:** High in protein, low in sodium and phosphorus.

Turkey and Vegetable Skillet

- **P.T.:** 25 mins
- **Ingr.:** 1 lb ground turkey, 1 cup diced bell peppers, 1 cup diced zucchini, 1 onion (chopped), 1 tsp garlic powder, 1 tbsp olive oil.
- **Procedure:** Cook turkey and vegetables in olive oil, season with garlic powder.
- **Tips:** Top with fresh parsley for added flavor.
- **N.I.:** Lean protein source, rich in vitamins, low in potassium.

Beef Stir-Fry with Broccoli

- **P.T.:** 20 mins
- **Ingr.:** 1 lb lean beef (sliced), 2 cups broccoli florets, 1 red bell pepper (sliced), sauce (low-sodium soy sauce, ginger, garlic).
- **Procedure:** Stir-fry beef, add vegetables and sauce. Cook until veggies are crisp-tender.
- **Tips:** Serve over brown rice or quinoa.
- **N.I.:** High in iron, low in sodium.

Pork Tenderloin with Apple Sauce

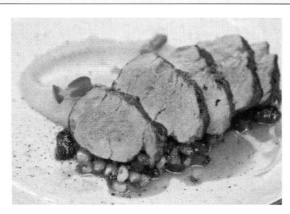

- **P.T.:** 45 mins
- **Ingr.:** 1 pork tenderloin, 2 apples (sliced), 1 tsp cinnamon, 1 tbsp honey, 1 tbsp olive oil.
- **Procedure:** Roast pork with apples, cinnamon, and honey until cooked.
- **Tips:** Slice pork and serve with a side of the cooked apples.
- **N.I.:** Low in phosphorus, high in protein.

Balsamic Glazed Chicken Salad

- **P.T.:** 20 mins
- **Ingr.:** 2 chicken breasts, mixed greens, cherry tomatoes, balsamic vinegar, 1 tbsp olive oil, black pepper.
- **Procedure:** Grill chicken, slice and serve over salad greens and tomatoes. Drizzle with balsamic vinegar and olive oil.
- **Tips:** Add sliced strawberries for a sweet touch.
- **N.I.:** High in protein, low in sodium, refreshing and light.

Poultry-Based Dishes: Versatile and Healthy

Herb-Roasted Chicken with Root Vegetables

- **P.T.:** 1 hour 15 mins
- **Ingr.:** 1 whole chicken, 2 carrots (chopped), 2 parsnips (chopped), 1 onion (quartered), 2 tbsp olive oil, 1 tsp rosemary, 1 tsp thyme.
- **Procedure:** Rub chicken with herbs and olive oil. Roast with vegetables until chicken is cooked and veggies are tender.
- **Tips:** Let the chicken rest for 10 minutes before carving.
- **N.I.:** Rich in protein, low in sodium, and phosphorus.

Lemon Garlic Turkey Breast

- **P.T.:** 1 hour
- **Ingr.:** 1 turkey breast, juice of 1 lemon, 3 cloves garlic (minced), 1 tbsp olive oil, black pepper to taste.
- **Procedure:** Marinate turkey in lemon, garlic, and olive oil. Bake until fully cooked.
- **Tips:** Slice thinly and serve with a side of steamed green beans.
- **N.I.:** Low in potassium, high in lean protein.

Spiced Chicken Kebabs

- **P.T.:** 45 mins (includes marinating time)
- **Ingr.:** 2 chicken breasts (cubed), 1 bell pepper (cubed), 1 onion (cubed), marinade (low-sodium yogurt, cumin, paprika), wooden skewers.
- **Procedure:** Marinate chicken, thread onto skewers with veggies. Grill until cooked.
- **Tips:** Serve with a yogurt-based dipping sauce.
- **N.I.:** High in protein, low in sodium.

Chicken and Vegetable Stir-Fry

- **P.T.:** 25 mins
- **Ingr.:** 2 chicken breasts (sliced), 2 cups mixed vegetables (broccoli, carrots, bell peppers), sauce (1 tbsp low-sodium soy sauce, ginger, garlic), 1 tbsp sesame oil.
- **Procedure:** Stir-fry chicken and veggies in sesame oil. Add sauce and cook until vegetables are crisp-tender.
- **Tips:** Serve over a small portion of brown rice.
- **N.I.:** Rich in vitamins, low in phosphorus.

Turkey and Spinach Meatballs

- **P.T.:** 35 mins
- **Ingr.:** 1 lb ground turkey, 1 cup spinach (finely chopped), 1 egg, 1/4 cup breadcrumbs, 1 tsp garlic powder, 1 tbsp olive oil.
- **Procedure:** Mix ingredients, form into meatballs. Bake until cooked through.
- **Tips:** Pair with a low-sodium tomato sauce and whole wheat pasta.
- **N.I.:** High in iron, moderate in protein, low in sodium.

Slow-Cooked Meals for Depth of Flavor

Savory Beef Stew

- **P.T.:** 8 hours (slow cooker)
- **Ingr.:** 1 lb lean beef cubes, 3 carrots (sliced), 2 potatoes (cubed), 1 onion (chopped), 4 cups low-sodium beef broth, 1 tsp thyme, 1 tbsp olive oil.
- **Procedure:** Brown beef in olive oil, transfer to slow cooker with all ingredients. Cook on low for 8 hours.
- **Tips:** Thicken with a cornstarch slurry if desired.
- **N.I.:** High in protein, low in sodium and phosphorus.

Chicken Cacciatore

- **P.T.:** 6 hours (slow cooker)
- **Ingr.:** 4 chicken thighs, 1 can no-salt-added diced tomatoes, 1 bell pepper (sliced), 1 onion (sliced), 1 tsp oregano, 1 tbsp olive oil, garlic powder to taste.
- **Procedure:** Place chicken, vegetables, tomatoes, and spices in slow cooker. Cook on low for 6 hours.
- **Tips:** Serve with whole grain pasta or brown rice.
- **N.I.:** Low in potassium, moderate in sodium.

Pork Loin with Apples and Onions

- **P.T.:** 7 hours (slow cooker)
- **Ingr.:** 1 pork loin, 2 apples (sliced), 2 onions (sliced), 1 tsp cinnamon, 1/4 cup apple cider, 1 tbsp olive oil.
- **Procedure:** Brown pork loin, place in slow cooker with apples, onions, cinnamon, and cider. Cook on low for 7 hours.
- **Tips:** Perfect for a fall or winter meal.
- **N.I.:** Low in sodium, high in protein.

Turkey Chili

- **P.T.:** 8 hours (slow cooker)
- **Ingr.:** 1 lb ground turkey, 1 can low-sodium kidney beans (drained), 1 can no-salt-added diced tomatoes, 1 onion (chopped), 1 bell pepper (chopped), chili powder to taste.
- **Procedure:** Cook turkey, combine in slow cooker with beans, tomatoes, onion, pepper, and spices. Cook on low for 8 hours.
- **Tips:** Top with a dollop of low-fat sour cream.
- **N.I.:** High in protein, fiber, and low in potassium.

Balsamic Braised Short Ribs

- **P.T.:** 7 hours (slow cooker)
- **Ingr.:** 4 beef short ribs, 1/4 cup balsamic vinegar, 1 onion (chopped), 2 cloves garlic (minced), 4 cups low-sodium beef broth, 1 tbsp olive oil, black pepper to taste.
- **Procedure:** Sear ribs, place in slow cooker with vinegar, onion, garlic, broth. Cook on low for 7 hours.
- **Tips:** Serve with mashed cauliflower or steamed greens.
- **N.I.:** Rich in flavor, low in sodium.

Chapter 7: Fish and Seafood Specialties

The Benefits of Omega-3s in Kidney Health

Garlic-Lemon Baked Salmon

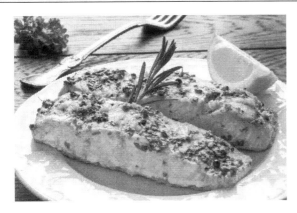

- **P.T.:** 25 mins

- **Ingr.:** 2 salmon fillets, 1 tbsp olive oil, 2 cloves garlic (minced), juice of 1 lemon, black pepper to taste.
- **Procedure:** Marinate salmon in olive oil, garlic, lemon juice, and pepper. Bake until flaky.
- **Tips:** Serve with a side of steamed asparagus.
- **N.I.:** High in omega-3 fatty acids, low in phosphorus.

Herb-Crusted Cod

- **P.T.:** 20 mins
- **Ingr.:** 2 cod fillets, 1/4 cup whole wheat breadcrumbs, 1 tsp dried herbs (parsley, dill), 1 tbsp olive oil, lemon wedges for serving.

- **Procedure:** Coat cod in breadcrumbs and herbs, drizzle with olive oil. Bake until golden.
- **Tips:** Squeeze fresh lemon over cooked cod for added zest.
- **N.I.:** Low in sodium, high in protein.

Grilled Tuna Steaks with Olive Tapenade

- **P.T.:** 30 mins
- **Ingr.:** 2 tuna steaks, 1/2 cup chopped olives, 1 tbsp capers, 1 clove garlic (minced), 2 tbsp olive oil.
- **Procedure:** Grill tuna steaks. Mix olives, capers, garlic, and olive oil for tapenade. Serve over tuna.
- **Tips:** Ideal for a high-protein meal; avoid overcooking the tuna
- **N.I.:** Rich in omega-3s, low in potassium.

Baked Trout with Almond Flakes

- **P.T.:** 25 mins
- **Ingr.:** 2 trout fillets, 1/4 cup sliced almonds, 1 tbsp butter, lemon zest, parsley for garnish.
- **Procedure:** Place trout in baking dish, top with almonds, dot with butter and lemon zest. Bake until cooked.
- **Tips:** Garnish with fresh parsley for a colorful finish.
- **N.I.:** High in healthy fats, moderate in phosphorus.

Shrimp and Spinach Salad

- **P.T.:** 20 mins
- **Ingr.:** 1 lb shrimp (peeled and deveined), 4 cups baby spinach, 1 avocado (sliced), dressing (olive oil, lemon juice, garlic powder).
- **Procedure:** Sauté shrimp, serve over spinach and avocado. Drizzle with dressing.
- **Tips:** Chilled shrimp can also be used for a refreshing touch.
- **N.I.:** High in protein, low in sodium, rich in antioxidants.

Grilled and Baked Fish Recipes

Mediterranean Grilled Mackerel

- **P.T.:** 20 mins
- **Ingr.:** 2 mackerel fillets, 1 lemon (sliced), 2 tbsp olive oil, 1 tsp dried oregano, black pepper to taste.
- **Procedure:** Marinate mackerel with lemon, olive oil, oregano, and pepper. Grill until cooked.
- **Tips:** Serve with a side of grilled vegetables.
- **N.I.:** High in omega-3s, low in sodium.

Baked Haddock with Herb Crust

- **P.T.:** 30 mins
- **Ingr.:** 2 haddock fillets, 1/4 cup whole wheat breadcrumbs, 1 tbsp chopped parsley, 1 tsp lemon zest, 1 tbsp olive oil.
- **Procedure:** Combine breadcrumbs, parsley, lemon zest. Coat fillets, drizzle with oil, bake.
- **Tips:** Perfect when paired with a fresh garden salad.
- **N.I.:** Low in phosphorus, high in protein.

Honey-Glazed Salmon

- **P.T.:** 25 mins
- **Ingr.:** 2 salmon fillets, 2 tbsp honey, 1 tbsp low-sodium soy sauce, 1 tsp garlic powder, 1 tbsp olive oil.
- **Procedure:** Mix honey, soy sauce, garlic; brush on salmon. Bake until glaze is caramelized.
- **Tips:** Garnish with sesame seeds and green onions.
- **N.I.:** Rich in omega-3s, low in sodium.

Citrus Tilapia en Papillote

- **P.T.:** 30 mins
- **Ingr.:** 2 tilapia fillets, 1 orange (sliced), 1 lemon (sliced), 1 lime (sliced), 1 tbsp olive oil, herbs (dill, parsley).
- **Procedure:** Place fillets on parchment paper, top with citrus slices, herbs, drizzle with oil. Seal and bake.
- **Tips:** This cooking method keeps the fish moist.
- **N.I.:** Low in fat, high in vitamin C.

Grilled Shrimp Skewers with Lime

- **P.T.:** 15 mins
- **Ingr.:** 1 lb shrimp (peeled, deveined), 2 limes (juiced), 1 tbsp olive oil, 1 tsp paprika, wooden skewers.
- **Procedure:** Marinate shrimp in lime juice, olive oil, paprika. Thread on skewers, grill.
- **Tips:** Serve with a lime wedge for extra zest.
- **N.I.:** High in protein, low in potassium.

Kidney-Friendly Seafood Pasta and Risottos

Shrimp and Asparagus Risotto

- **P.T.:** 40 mins
- **Ingr.:** 1 cup Arborio rice, 1 lb shrimp (peeled and deveined), 2 cups chopped asparagus, 1 onion (chopped), 4 cups low-sodium vegetable broth, 1 tbsp olive oil, lemon zest.
- **Procedure:** Sauté onion, add rice. Gradually add broth, stirring. Add asparagus, shrimp. Cook until shrimp are done. Stir in lemon zest.
- **Tips:** Garnish with parsley for a fresh finish.
- **N.I.:** High in protein, low in sodium.

Seafood Pasta Primavera

- **P.T.:** 30 mins
- **Ingr.:** 8 oz whole wheat pasta, 1 cup mixed seafood (shrimp, scallops), 2 cups mixed vegetables (zucchini, bell peppers), 1 can no-salt-added diced tomatoes, 1 tsp garlic powder, 1 tbsp olive oil.
- **Procedure:** Cook pasta, set aside. Sauté seafood and vegetables, add tomatoes and garlic powder. Toss with pasta.
- **Tips:** Serve with a sprinkle of Parmesan, if desired.
- **N.I.:** Balanced in carbs and protein, low in potassium.

Lemon-Garlic Scallops over Linguine

- **P.T.:** 25 mins
- **Ingr.:** 1 lb scallops, 8 oz whole wheat linguine, 2 cloves garlic (minced), juice of 1 lemon, 2 tbsp parsley (chopped), 1 tbsp olive oil.
- **Procedure:** Cook linguine. Sauté scallops with garlic, lemon juice. Serve over linguine, garnish with parsley.
- **Tips:** Avoid overcooking the scallops to keep them tender.
- **N.I.:** High in omega-3 fatty acids, low in sodium.

Tuna and Olive Spaghetti

- **P.T.:** 20 mins
- **Ingr.:** 8 oz whole wheat spaghetti, 1 can no-salt-added tuna (drained), 1/4 cup chopped olives, 1 tbsp capers, 2 tbsp olive oil, 1 tsp dried oregano.
- **Procedure:** Cook spaghetti. Mix tuna, olives, capers, olive oil, oregano. Toss with spaghetti.
- **Tips:** Add a squeeze of lemon for extra zest.
- **N.I.:** Rich in protein, low in phosphorus.

Creamy Shrimp and Mushroom Fettuccine

- **P.T.:** 30 mins
- **Ingr.:** 8 oz whole wheat fettuccine, 1 lb shrimp, 1 cup sliced mushrooms, 1 cup low-fat milk, 2 tbsp flour, 1 tbsp butter, 1 tsp parsley.
- **Procedure:** Cook fettuccine. Sauté shrimp, set aside. Cook mushrooms in butter, add flour, slowly add milk to create a sauce. Add shrimp, toss with pasta.
- **Tips:** Garnish with parsley and black pepper.
- **N.I.:** Low in sodium, high in flavor.

Chapter 8: Sides and Snacks

Vegetable Sides: Steamed, Roasted, and Beyond

Garlic Roasted Brussels Sprouts

- **P.T.:** 25 mins
- **Ingr.:** 2 cups Brussels sprouts (halved), 2 cloves garlic (minced), 1 tbsp olive oil, black pepper to taste.
- **Procedure:** Toss Brussels sprouts with garlic, olive oil, and pepper. Roast until crispy.
- **Tips:** Add a sprinkle of Parmesan cheese for extra flavor.
- **N.I.:** Low in sodium, high in vitamins C and K.

Herbed Carrot and Parsnip Fries

- **P.T.:** 30 mins
- **Ingr.:** 2 carrots, 2 parsnips (cut into sticks), 1 tsp dried rosemary, 1 tsp dried thyme, 1 tbsp olive oil.
- **Procedure:** Toss carrots and parsnips with oil and herbs. Bake until golden and tender.
- **Tips:** Perfect as a healthy alternative to traditional fries.
- **N.I.:** High in fiber, low in potassium.

Steamed Green Beans with Almonds

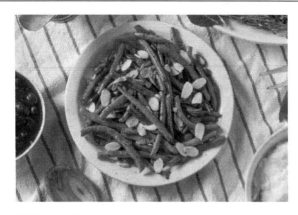

- **P.T.:** 15 mins
- **Ingr.:** 2 cups green beans (trimmed), 1/4 cup slivered almonds, 1 tbsp lemon juice, 1 tbsp olive oil.
- **Procedure:** Steam green beans until tender-crisp. Toss with almonds, lemon juice, and olive oil.
- **Tips:** Can be served warm or cold as a salad.
- **N.I.:** Low in sodium, rich in healthy fats.

Spicy Cauliflower Roast

- **P.T.:** 35 mins
- **Ingr.:** 1 head cauliflower (cut into florets), 1 tsp paprika, 1/2 tsp garlic powder, 1 tbsp olive oil, black pepper to taste.
- **Procedure:** Toss cauliflower with spices and oil. Roast until tender and slightly charred.
- **Tips:** Adjust the spice level according to your preference.
- **N.I.:** Low in phosphorus, high in vitamin C.

Balsamic Glazed Beetroot

- **P.T.:** 1 hour
- **Ingr.:** 4 beetroots (peeled and sliced), 2 tbsp balsamic vinegar, 1 tbsp olive oil, 1 tsp thyme.
- **Procedure:** Roast beetroots with oil and thyme. Drizzle with balsamic vinegar in the last 10 minutes.
- **Tips:** Serve as a colorful addition to any meal.
- **N.I.:** High in antioxidants, low in sodium.

Snacks: Quick Bites for Energy and Health

Cucumber and Hummus Roll-Ups

- **P.T.:** 15 mins
- **Ingr.:** 1 cucumber (sliced lengthwise), 1 cup low-sodium hummus, 1/4 cup red bell pepper (finely diced), fresh dill for garnish.
- **Procedure:** Spread hummus on cucumber slices, add bell pepper, roll up. Garnish with dill.
- **Tips:** Chill before serving for a refreshing snack.
- **N.I.:** Low in potassium, high in fiber.

Avocado and Tomato Bruschetta

- **P.T.:** 10 mins
- **Ingr.:** 1 ripe avocado (mashed), 1 tomato (diced), 2 tbsp chopped onion, whole grain toast, lemon juice, black pepper.
- **Procedure:** Mix avocado, tomato, onion, lemon juice. Spoon onto toast, season with pepper.
- **Tips:** Ideal for a quick and nutritious breakfast or snack.
- **N.I.:** Rich in healthy fats, low in sodium.

Baked Kale Chips

- **P.T.:** 20 mins
- **Ingr.:** 2 cups kale leaves (torn), 1 tbsp olive oil, garlic powder, black pepper.
- **Procedure:** Toss kale in oil, season. Bake until crisp.
- **Tips:** Store in an airtight container to maintain crispness.
- **N.I.:** High in vitamins A and C, low in sodium.

Carrot and Almond Butter Pinwheels

- **P.T.:** 10 mins
- **Ingr.:** 1 large carrot (shaved into ribbons), 2 tbsp almond butter, whole grain tortillas.
- **Procedure:** Spread almond butter on tortillas, lay carrot ribbons, roll up and slice.
- **Tips:** A crunchy and satisfying snack, great for on-the-go.
- **N.I.:** Good source of beta-carotene, low in phosphorus.

Roasted Chickpeas

- **P.T.:** 30 mins
- **Ingr.:** 1 can low-sodium chickpeas (drained and rinsed), 1 tbsp olive oil, 1 tsp smoked paprika, black pepper.
- **Procedure:** Toss chickpeas with oil and spices. Roast until crispy.
- **Tips:** Experiment with different spices for variety.
- **N.I.:** High in protein and fiber, low in sodium.

Grains and Legumes: Safe and Satisfying Options

Quinoa Tabbouleh

- **P.T.:** 20 mins
- **Ingr.:** 1 cup cooked quinoa, 1 cup chopped parsley, 1/2 cup chopped tomatoes, 1/4 cup chopped mint, 2 tbsp lemon juice, 1 tbsp olive oil.
- **Procedure:** Mix quinoa with parsley, tomatoes, mint. Dress with lemon juice and olive oil.
- **Tips:** Chill before serving for flavors to meld.
- **N.I.:** High in protein, low in sodium, gluten-free.

Lentil and Veggie Stew

- **P.T.:** 45 mins
- **Ingr.:** 1 cup green lentils, 2 carrots (chopped), 2 celery stalks (chopped), 1 onion (chopped), 4 cups low-sodium vegetable broth, 1 tsp cumin.
- **Procedure:** Simmer lentils, vegetables, and cumin in broth until lentils are tender.
- **Tips:** Serve with a slice of whole grain bread.
- **N.I.:** Rich in fiber, low in potassium.

Black Bean and Corn Salad

- **P.T.:** 15 mins
- **Ingr.:** 1 can low-sodium black beans (drained, rinsed), 1 cup corn, 1 diced red bell pepper, 1/4 cup chopped cilantro, 2 tbsp lime juice, 1 tbsp olive oil.
- **Procedure:** Combine beans, corn, bell pepper, cilantro. Dress with lime juice and olive oil.
- **Tips:** Perfect as a side dish or a light lunch.
- **N.I.:** High in plant-based protein, low in sodium.

Barley and Mushroom Pilaf

- **P.T.:** 30 mins
- **Ingr.:** 1 cup pearl barley, 2 cups sliced mushrooms, 1 onion (chopped), 4 cups low-sodium vegetable broth, 1 tsp thyme, 1 tbsp olive oil.
- **Procedure:** Sauté onion and mushrooms, add barley, broth, thyme. Simmer until barley is tender.
- **Tips:** Fluff with a fork before serving.
- **N.I.:** Low in sodium, high in soluble fiber.

Chapter 9: Desserts and Sweet Treats

Managing Sugar and Sweetness

Managing sugar and sweetness in desserts, particularly for individuals on a renal diet, necessitates a thoughtful approach that goes beyond just satisfying sweet cravings. This comprehensive look at dessert crafting aims to highlight ways to indulge responsibly, ensuring that each sweet treat aligns with dietary needs while still delighting the taste buds.

Navigating the landscape of sugar consumption is pivotal for those mindful of their renal health. The human palate naturally craves sweetness, yet in the context of renal wellness, this craving must be met with careful consideration. Excessive sugar intake is linked with adverse health effects, including exacerbating conditions like diabetes, which directly impacts renal function. Additionally, high sugar levels can contribute to weight gain and elevated blood pressure, further burdening the kidneys.

The culinary world is abundant with natural sweeteners that offer a wholesome alternative to refined sugars. Sweeteners such as honey, maple syrup, and agave nectar, though requiring moderate use, provide a gentler impact on the body's sugar levels. Stevia, a naturally derived sweetener, stands out as a calorie-free option that does not raise blood sugar levels, making it an ideal choice for those needing to closely manage their sugar intake.

Fruits play a quintessential role in naturally sweetening desserts. They come packed not only with sugars but also with essential fibers, vitamins, and minerals, creating a balanced nutritional profile. Using fruits like ripe bananas, apples, or berries can bring natural sweetness to various desserts. For example, mashed bananas can serve as a perfect sweetening agent in baking, while apple sauce can replace sugar in recipes, adding both sweetness and moisture.

Mindful indulgence is key when incorporating sweets into a renal-friendly diet. Portion control is essential; it helps regulate sugar intake and maintain a healthy weight. Opting for smaller dessert portions or creating bite-sized treats can effectively keep sugar consumption in check while still allowing for a satisfying experience.

Renal diet-compliant desserts require innovation and creativity. Avocado-based mousse flavored with cocoa powder and honey, or chia seed puddings made with almond milk and infused with natural flavors like vanilla or cinnamon, offer delightful alternatives to traditional sweets. These recipes fulfill the desire for a decadent dessert while fitting within the constraints of a renal diet.

Awareness and knowledge are crucial in managing sugar within a renal-friendly diet. Understanding different types of sugars and sweeteners, recognizing hidden sugars in processed foods, and being aware of the glycemic impact of various sweetening options can empower individuals to make informed dessert choices.

Fruit-Based Desserts: Natural and Nutritious

Baked Cinnamon Apples

- **P.T.:** 30 mins
- **Ingr.:** 4 apples (cored and sliced), 2 tsp cinnamon, 1 tbsp honey, 1/4 cup walnuts (chopped).
- **Procedure:** Place apple slices in a baking dish. Sprinkle with cinnamon and honey, top with walnuts. Bake until tender.
- **Tips:** Serve warm with a dollop of low-fat Greek yogurt.
- **N.I.:** Low in sodium, high in fiber.

Berry Salad with Mint

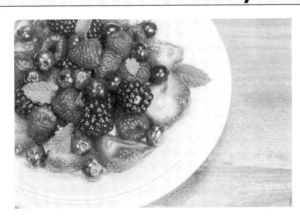

- **P.T.:** 10 mins
- **Ingr.:** 2 cups mixed berries (strawberries, blueberries, raspberries), 1 tbsp fresh mint (chopped), 1 tsp lemon zest, 1 tbsp orange juice.
- **Procedure:** Toss berries with mint, lemon zest, and orange juice.
- **Tips:** Chill before serving for a refreshing dessert.
- **N.I.:** Rich in antioxidants, low in potassium.

Peach and Yogurt Parfait

- **P.T.:** 15 mins
- **Ingr.:** 2 peaches (sliced), 1 cup low-fat Greek yogurt, 2 tbsp granola, 1 tsp honey.
- **Procedure:** Layer yogurt, peaches, and granola in a glass. Drizzle with honey.
- **Tips:** Perfect for a quick and healthy snack or dessert.
- **N.I.:** High in protein, low in sodium.

Grilled Pineapple with Cinnamon

- **P.T.:** 15 mins
- **Ingr.:** 1 pineapple (sliced), 2 tsp cinnamon, 1 tbsp honey.
- **Procedure:** Grill pineapple slices, sprinkle with cinnamon, drizzle with honey.
- **Tips:** Serve with a scoop of low-fat vanilla ice cream.
- **N.I.:** Low in phosphorus, natural sweetness.

Banana and Almond Butter Bites

- **P.T.:** 10 mins
- **Ingr.:** 2 bananas (sliced), 1/4 cup almond butter, 1/4 cup dark chocolate chips (melted).
- **Procedure:** Spread almond butter on banana slices, drizzle with melted chocolate.
- **Tips:** Freeze for a cool treat.
- **N.I.:** High in potassium, suitable in moderation.

Watermelon and Feta Salad

- **P.T.:** 10 mins
- **Ingr.:** 2 cups watermelon (cubed), 1/2 cup feta cheese (crumbled), 1 tbsp balsamic glaze, fresh basil.
- **Procedure:** Toss watermelon with feta, drizzle with balsamic glaze, garnish with basil.
- **Tips:** A unique combination of sweet and savory.
- **N.I.:** Low in sodium, refreshing.

Kiwi and Strawberry Popsicles

- **P.T.:** 4 hours (freezing time)
- **Ingr.:** 3 kiwis (sliced), 1 cup strawberries (sliced), 1 cup coconut water.
- **Procedure:** Fill popsicle molds with kiwi and strawberry slices, pour in coconut water. Freeze until solid.
- **Tips:** A hydrating and fruity snack for hot days.
- **N.I.:** Rich in vitamin C, low in phosphorus.

Baked Goods: Kidney-Safe Indulgences

Almond Flour Blueberry Muffins

- **P.T.:** 35 mins
- **Ingr.:** 2 cups almond flour, 1/2 cup fresh blueberries, 2 eggs, 1/4 cup honey, 1 tsp vanilla extract, 1 tsp baking powder.
- **Procedure:** Mix ingredients, fold in blueberries. Pour into muffin tins, bake until golden.
- **Tips:** Ideal for a kidney-friendly breakfast or snack.
- **N.I.:** Low in sodium, high in healthy fats.

Carrot and Walnut Cake

- **P.T.:** 50 mins
- **Ingr.:** 1 1/2 cups whole wheat flour, 1 cup grated carrots, 1/2 cup chopped walnuts, 2 eggs, 1/2 cup applesauce, 1/4 cup vegetable oil, 1 tsp cinnamon.
- **Procedure:** Combine ingredients, pour into a cake tin, bake. Optional: Top with low-fat cream cheese frosting.
- **Tips:** Moist and flavorful, great for celebrations.
- **N.I.:** Rich in fiber, lower in sugar.

Oatmeal Banana Cookies

- **P.T.:** 25 mins
- **Ingr.:** 2 ripe bananas (mashed), 1 cup rolled oats, 1/4 cup raisins, 1 tsp cinnamon, 1 tbsp honey.
- **Procedure:** Mix ingredients, spoon onto baking sheet, bake until set.
- **Tips:** Perfect for a quick, healthy snack.
- **N.I.:** Low in sodium, natural sweetness from bananas.

Lemon Poppy Seed Loaf

- **P.T.:** 55 mins
- **Ingr.:** 1 1/2 cups all-purpose flour, 1/2 cup sugar, 1/4 cup poppy seeds, 2 eggs, 1/2 cup unsalted butter, juice and zest of 1 lemon.
- **Procedure:** Cream butter and sugar, add eggs, flour, lemon, poppy seeds. Bake in loaf pan.
- **Tips:** Glaze with a mix of lemon juice and powdered sugar for extra zest.
- **N.I.:** Moderate in potassium delightful lemon flavor.

Peach and Ginger Crisp

- **P.T.:** 40 mins
- **Ingr.:** 4 peaches (sliced), 1/2 cup rolled oats, 1/4 cup almond flour, 1/4 cup brown sugar, 1 tsp ground ginger, 1/4 cup unsalted butter.
- **Procedure:** Layer peaches in dish. Mix oats, flour, sugar, ginger, butter. Crumble over peaches, bake.
- **Tips:** Serve warm with a scoop of low-fat ice cream.
- **N.I.:** Low in sodium, natural fruit sugars.

Chocolate Zucchini Bread

- **P.T.:** 1 hour
- **Ingr.:** 1 1/2 cups whole wheat flour, 1 cup grated zucchini, 1/2 cup cocoa powder, 2 eggs, 1/2 cup vegetable oil, 1/2 cup sugar, 1 tsp vanilla.
- **Procedure:** Mix all ingredients, pour into loaf pan, bake until a toothpick comes out clean.
- **Tips:** Great way to sneak in veggies for kids.
- **N.I.:** Rich in antioxidants, lower in phosphorus.

Apple and Cinnamon Scones

- **P.T.:** 30 mins
- **Ingr.:** 2 cups all-purpose flour, 1/2 cup diced apples, 1/3 cup sugar, 1/2 cup unsalted butter, 1 tsp cinnamon, 1 tsp baking powder.
- **Procedure:** Combine ingredients, form into scones, bake until golden.
- **Tips:** Delicious when served with a cup of herbal tea.
- **N.I.:** Low in sodium, indulgent yet kidney-friendly.

Chapter 10: Beverages and Smoothies

Hydration and Kidney Health: What to Know

Hydration holds a pivotal role in maintaining kidney health, acting as a cornerstone for those managing their renal diet. The kidneys, sophisticated in their function, are responsible for filtering and removing waste products from the body. Adequate hydration is essential in facilitating these processes, ensuring that the kidneys function efficiently.

The essence of hydration goes beyond merely drinking water; it encompasses understanding the right balance and the types of fluids beneficial for renal health. Water is, undoubtedly, the most kidney-friendly drink, providing a pure and straightforward means to stay hydrated without any added sugars, sodium, or harmful additives. The recommended daily water intake can vary based on individual health needs, lifestyle, and even climate. It's crucial for those with kidney concerns to consult healthcare professionals to determine their optimal water intake.

In addition to water, other beverages can contribute positively to hydration while being mindful of kidney health. For instance, certain herbal teas offer a kidney-friendly alternative to caffeinated drinks. These herbal infusions, free from caffeine, can aid in hydration while providing a variety of flavors to enjoy. Beverages like cranberry juice, when chosen in their unsweetened forms, can be beneficial. They contain compounds that may help prevent urinary tract infections, a common concern for those with kidney issues.

However, not all fluids are created equal when it comes to kidney health. Beverages high in sugars, artificial sweeteners, or caffeine can pose challenges. Excessive sugar can lead to health problems such as obesity or diabetes, both of which are risk factors for kidney disease. Artificial sweeteners, while helpful in reducing sugar intake, should be used cautiously and in moderation. Caffeinated drinks, though they can contribute to overall fluid intake, should be consumed in limited quantities as they can potentially increase blood pressure, a factor that can stress the kidneys.

Alcoholic beverages are another category that requires careful consideration. Alcohol can be dehydrating and, when consumed in excess, can lead to liver disease, another contributor to kidney stress. Moderation is key, and in some cases, abstention, depending on individual health status.

Hydration also extends to the foods we eat. Many fruits and vegetables have high water content and can contribute significantly to overall fluid intake. Foods like cucumbers, zucchinis, watermelons, and oranges are not only hydrating but also provide essential vitamins and minerals.

Herbal Teas and Infusions

Mint and Lemon Balm Tea

- **P.T.:** 10 mins
- **Ingr.:** A handful of fresh mint leaves, a few lemon balm leaves, boiling water.
- **Procedure:** Steep mint and lemon balm in boiling water for 5-10 minutes.
- **Tips:** Enjoy hot or chilled with a slice of lemon for extra zest.
- **N.I.:** Caffeine-free, aids in digestion, low in potassium.

Chamomile and Lavender Soothe

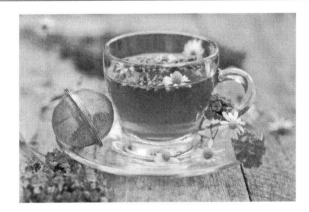

- **P.T.:** 10 mins
- **Ingr.:** 1 tbsp dried chamomile flowers, 1 tsp dried lavender buds, boiling water.
- **Procedure:** Combine chamomile and lavender, steep in boiling water for 10 minutes.
- **Tips:** A calming tea, perfect before bedtime.
- **N.I.:** Caffeine-free, relaxing properties.

Ginger and Turmeric Infusion

- **P.T.:** 15 mins
- **Ingr.:** 1-inch fresh ginger (sliced), 1/2 tsp turmeric powder, 1 tsp honey, boiling water.
- **Procedure:** Steep ginger and turmeric in boiling water, strain and add honey.
- **Tips:** Can be enjoyed hot or cold; great for anti-inflammatory benefits.
- **N.I.:** Low in sodium, aids in digestion.

Rosehip and Hibiscus Delight

- **P.T.:** 10 mins
- **Ingr.:** 1 tbsp dried rosehips, 1 tbsp dried hibiscus flowers, boiling water.
- **Procedure:** Steep rosehips and hibiscus in boiling water for 10 minutes.
- **Tips:** Serve chilled with a splash of sparkling water for a refreshing drink.
- **N.I.:** High in vitamin C, caffeine-free.

Cinnamon and Apple Warmth

- **P.T.:** 10 mins
- **Ingr.:** 1 cinnamon stick, 1/2 apple (sliced), boiling water.
- **Procedure:** Combine cinnamon and apple in boiling water, steep for 10 minutes.
- **Tips:** Ideal for colder months, can be sweetened with a touch of honey.
- **N.I.:** Caffeine-free, warming, low in potassium.

Nutritious Smoothies and Shakes

Berry Blast Kidney Care Smoothie

- **P.T.:** 10 mins
- **Ingr.:** 1/2 cup blueberries, 1/2 cup strawberries, 1 banana, 1 cup almond milk, 1 tbsp chia seeds.
- **Procedure:** Blend all ingredients until smooth.
- **Tips:** Add ice for a thicker smoothie.
- **N.I.:** Rich in antioxidants, low in potassium.

Green Goddess Renal Health Shake

- **P.T.:** 10 mins
- **Ingr.:** 1 cup spinach, 1/2 avocado, 1/2 apple, 1 cup coconut water, 1 tsp honey.
- **Procedure:** Combine all ingredients in a blender, blend until creamy.
- **Tips:** Adjust sweetness with more or less honey as desired.
- **N.I.:** High in healthy fats, moderate in potassium.

Pineapple and Cucumber Hydration Smoothie

- **P.T.:** 10 mins
- **Ingr.:** 1 cup pineapple (cubed), 1/2 cucumber (sliced), 1 cup water, juice of 1 lime.
- **Procedure:** Blend all ingredients until smooth.
- **Tips:** Serve chilled for a refreshing and hydrating drink.
- **N.I.:** Low in sodium, refreshing, and hydrating.

Protein Power Shake

- **P.T.:** 10 mins
- **Ingr.:** 1 scoop low-potassium protein powder, 1 cup almond milk, 1/2 banana, 1 tbsp almond butter, 1 tsp cinnamon.
- **Procedure:** Blend all ingredients until creamy.
- **Tips:** Ideal as a post-exercise shake or a breakfast smoothie.
- **N.I.:** High in protein, low in phosphorus.

Carrot and Ginger Wellness Smoothie

- **P.T.:** 10 mins
- **Ingr.:** 2 carrots (peeled and chopped), 1-inch ginger (peeled), 1 apple, 1 cup water, 1 tsp lemon juice.
- **Procedure:** Blend carrots, ginger, apple, and water until smooth. Add lemon juice.
- **Tips:** Great for boosting immunity and aiding digestion.
- **N.I.:** Rich in vitamins A and C, low in potassium.

Chapter 11: 5-Week Meal Plan

Week 1

Date	Breakfast	Lunch	Dinner	Snack 1	Snack 2
1	Avocado Zen Blend	Spinach and Strawberry Sensation	Garden Fresh Vegetable Soup	Lentil and Veggie Stew	Roasted Chickpeas
2	Avocado Egg Cups	Lentil and Roasted Veggie Toss	Mushroom and Barley Soup	Barley and Mushroom Pilaf	Black Bean and Corn Salad
3	Spinach and Mushroom Omelette	Spinach and Strawberry Sensation	Beef and Mushroom Stew	Baked Kale Chips	Berry Salad with Mint
4	Egg and Quinoa Breakfast Bowl	Cilantro Lime Dressing	Spicy Tomato and Chickpea Soup	Quinoa Tabbouleh	Lentil and Veggie Stew
5	Oat and Almond Flour Pancakes	Cilantro Lime Dressing	Chickpea and Spinach Curry	Peach and Yogurt Parfait	Banana and Almond Butter Bites
6	Protein Power Punch	Kale and Avocado Delight	Mushroom and Barley Soup	Quinoa Tabbouleh	Kiwi and Strawberry Popsicles
7	Buckwheat and Blueberry Pancakes	Crisp Arugula and Apple Salad	Spicy Tomato and Chickpea Stew	Roasted Chickpeas	Roasted Chickpeas

Week 2

Date	Breakfast	Lunch	Dinner	Snack 1	Snack 2
1	Tropical Turmeric Tango	Grilled Chicken and Quinoa Salad	Tomato Basil Soup	Avocado and Tomato Bruschetta	Barley and Mushroom Pilaf
2	Berry Almond Bliss	Tofu and Edamame Salad Bowl	Beef and Mushroom Stew	Roasted Chickpeas	Black Bean and Corn Salad
3	Quinoa Flour Waffles	Tofu and Edamame Salad Bowl	Moroccan Lentil and Vegetable Stew	Avocado and Tomato Bruschetta	Avocado and Tomato Bruschetta
4	Banana Chia Waffles	Lentil and Roasted Veggie Toss	Beef and Mushroom Stew	Carrot and Almond Butter Pinwheels	Black Bean and Corn Salad
5	Herbed Veggie Scramble	Chickpea and Avocado Medley	Moroccan Lentil and Vegetable Stew	Quinoa Tabbouleh	Roasted Chickpeas
6	Quinoa Flour Waffles	Lentil and Roasted Veggie Toss	Tomato Basil Soup	Lentil and Veggie Stew	Quinoa Tabbouleh
7	Berry Almond Bliss	Tofu and Edamame Salad Bowl	Winter Vegetable and Bean Stew	Carrot and Almond Butter Pinwheels	Quinoa Tabbouleh

Week 3

Date	Breakfast	Lunch	Dinner	Snack 1	Snack 2
1	Sweet Potato and Flaxseed Pancakes	Creamy Avocado Dressing	Butternut Squash and Lentil Soup	Carrot and Almond Butter Pinwheels	Carrot and Almond Butter Pinwheels
2	Sweet Potato and Flaxseed Pancakes	Lemon Herb Vinaigrette	Butternut Squash and Lentil Soup	Avocado and Tomato Bruschetta	Avocado and Tomato Bruschetta
3	Buckwheat and Blueberry Pancakes	Crisp Arugula and Apple Salad	Garden Fresh Vegetable Soup	Avocado and Tomato Bruschetta	Avocado and Tomato Bruschetta
4	Quinoa Flour Waffles	Raspberry Walnut Vinaigrette	Carrot and Ginger Puree Soup	Baked Kale Chips	Quinoa Tabbouleh
5	Banana Chia Waffles	Mixed Greens with Roasted Beetroot	Mushroom and Barley Soup	Lentil and Veggie Stew	Avocado and Tomato Bruschetta
6	Tropical Turmeric Tango	Raspberry Walnut Vinaigrette	Carrot and Ginger Puree Soup	Cucumber and Hummus Roll-Ups	Carrot and Almond Butter Pinwheels
7	Oat and Almond Flour Pancakes	Crisp Arugula and Apple Salad	Creamy Cauliflower and Garlic Soup	Quinoa Tabbouleh	Baked Kale Chips

Week 4

Date	Breakfast	Lunch	Dinner	Snack 1	Snack 2
1	Berry Almond Bliss	Chickpea and Avocado Medley	Creamy Cauliflower and Garlic Soup	Cucumber and Hummus Roll-Ups	Lentil and Veggie Stew
2	Avocado Zen Blend	Grilled Chicken and Quinoa Salad	Hearty Chicken and Barley Stew	Avocado and Tomato Bruschetta	Quinoa Tabbouleh
3	Green Detoxifier	Grilled Chicken and Quinoa Salad	Spicy Tomato and Chickpea Stew	Cucumber and Hummus Roll-Ups	Baked Kale Chips
4	Tropical Turmeric Tango	Tofu and Edamame Salad Bowl	Lentil and Spinach Broth	Cucumber and Hummus Roll-Ups	Roasted Chickpeas
5	Protein Power Punch	Creamy Avocado Dressing	Hearty Chicken and Barley Stew	Roasted Chickpeas	Lentil and Veggie Stew
6	Banana Chia Waffles	Creamy Avocado Dressing	Carrot and Ginger Puree Soup	Lentil and Veggie Stew	Lentil and Veggie Stew
7	Tropical Turmeric Tango	Grilled Chicken and Quinoa Salad	Spicy Tomato and Chickpea Stew	Baked Kale Chips	Avocado and Tomato Bruschetta

Week 5

Dat e	Breakfast	Lunch	Dinner	Snack 1	Snack 2
1	Buckwheat and Blueberry Pancakes	Mixed Greens with Roasted Beetroot	Garden Fresh Vegetable Soup	Lentil and Veggie Stew	Cucumber and Hummus Roll-Ups
2	Oat and Almond Flour Pancakes	Grilled Chicken and Quinoa Salad	Winter Vegetable and Bean Stew	Cucumber and Hummus Roll-Ups	Roasted Chickpeas
3	Buckwheat and Blueberry Pancakes	Tofu and Edamame Salad Bowl	Garden Fresh Vegetable Soup	Carrot and Almond Butter Pinwheels	Baked Kale Chips
4	Oat and Almond Flour Pancakes	Chickpea and Avocado Medley	Winter Vegetable and Bean Stew	Carrot and Almond Butter Pinwheels	Quinoa Tabbouleh
5	Sweet Potato and Flaxseed Pancakes	Tofu and Edamame Salad Bowl	Hearty Chicken and Barley Stew	Avocado and Tomato Bruschetta	Roasted Chickpeas
6	Banana Chia Waffles	Chickpea and Avocado Medley	Mushroom and Barley Soup	Baked Kale Chips	Quinoa Tabbouleh
7	Sweet Potato and Flaxseed Pancakes	Grilled Chicken and Quinoa Salad	Hearty Chicken and Barley Stew	Cucumber and Hummus Roll-Ups	Quinoa Tabbouleh

Index

Made in the USA
Columbia, SC
12 November 2024

46298837R00063